Viagra® Simplified

and other ED Medications

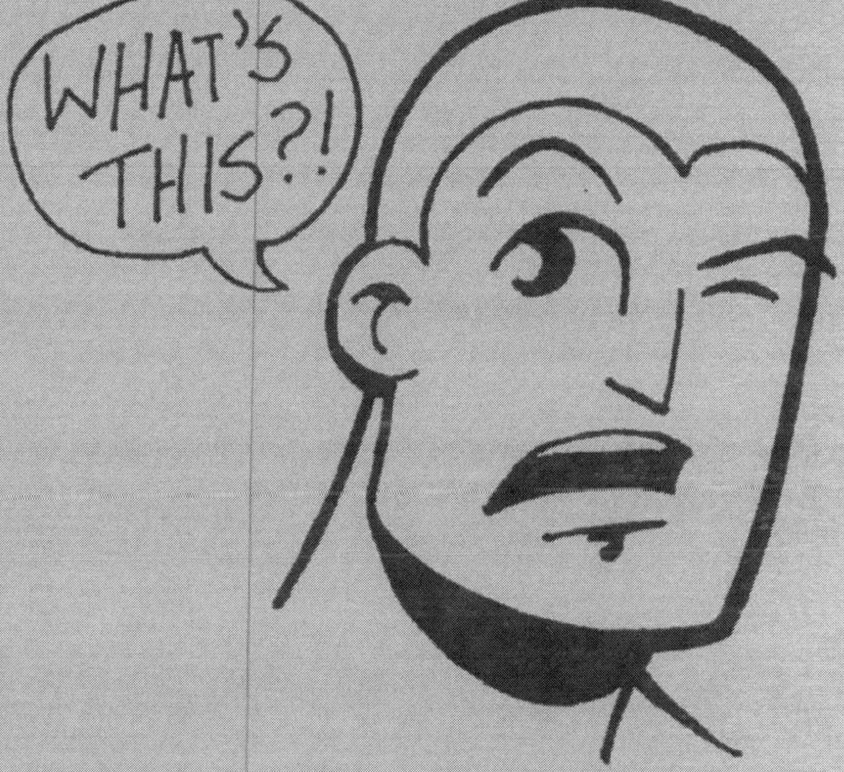

Viagra® Simplified
Understanding the Erection

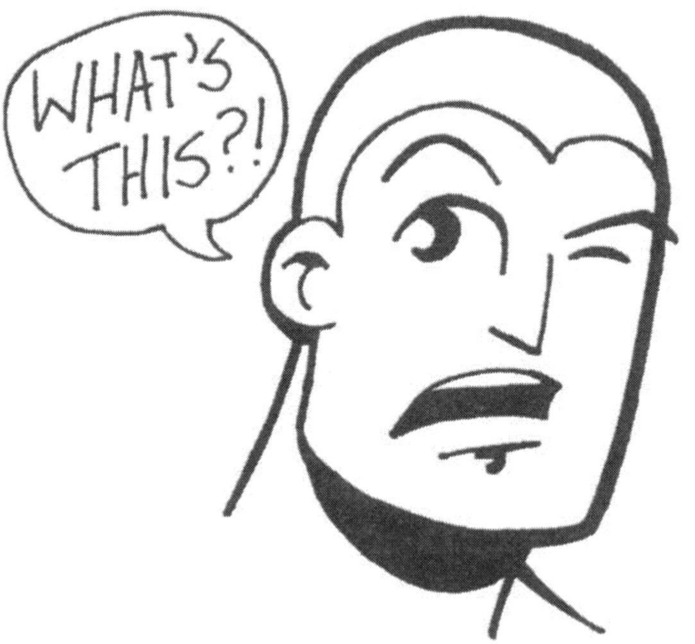

Introduction

Q: What do you get if you mix Viagra® and Rogaine

The answer to that joke is Don King. That joke is the level of understanding of the male erection. The erection is a subject which interests me as a middle age man and as a registered nurse. As someone who had written extensively on simplifications of medical topics, this seemed like a chance to write another book.

I met Ralph Zagha early one morning in the hospital. He was a new urologist who had just finished his residency at Harvard and Tufts University. We talked. I mentioned my idea for this book and here it is.

The goal of this book is to explain the physiology, pathophysiology and pharmacology of an erection. We will look at how an erection works, why sometimes problems occur and how medication and treatment can address them. If you understand how erections work, you can seek treatment more intelligently when they don't work.

This explanation will be aimed at many levels of understanding. It will be understandable to the person with no medical knowledge or experience. It will provide medically accurate facts. About 1/3 of the book will provide basic facts for consumers. Nothing will be difficult to understand.

For health care workers these facts will be surrounded by the other 2/3 of this book, the larger physiological context. That way you can understand those basic facts in the context of overall physiology. Again, nothing will be difficult to understand.

Viagra® - Levitra® - Cialis®

Viagra® was discovered by accident, fortunately not serious. While studying phosphodiesterase inhibitors for the treatment of high blood pressure, researchers at Pfizer noticed a persistent side effect, erections. Viagra (sildenafil) was approved by the FDA for erection problems in 1998.

Viagra® stormed into the American culture. Pfizer stock price soared. Millions of prescriptions were written. Jokes abounded. Talk show hosts had a new topic. Millions of dollars were spent on advertising. Former presidential candidate Robert Dole endorsed it on television as well as Nascar race driver Mark Martin who prominently displayed Viagra® on the hood of his racing car.

By 2003 Lilly came out with Cialis® (tadalafil) . This was followed by Bayer with Levitra® (vardenafil). All three are in the same pharmaceutical class, phosphodiesterase inhibitors. To those curious to understand how these drugs work we will explain the mechanism of action.

To avoid any lawsuits or charges of bias, or drug company payments, we will refer to these medications as phosphodiesterase inhibitors or abbreviated, PDE_5 inhibitors.

Anatomy of the Genito-Urinary System

All of our organs like our brain, heart, liver are surrounded by an ocean of fluids. Our body's normal function, even existence, depends on maintaining the proper ingredients in those fluids for nutrition, immunity, and waste exchange.

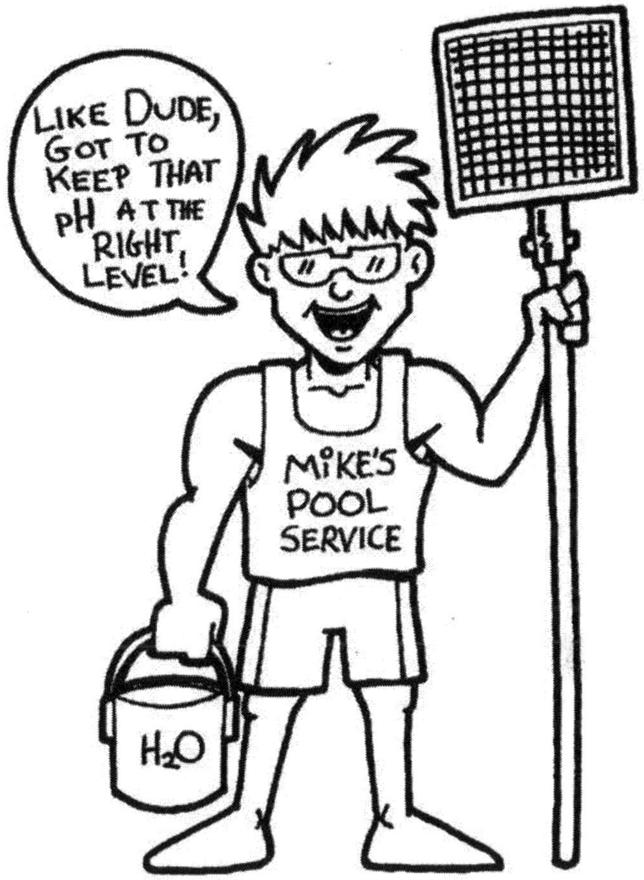

Let's say you lived your whole life in a swimming pool. You would depend on your pool cleaning service to keep the water correct.

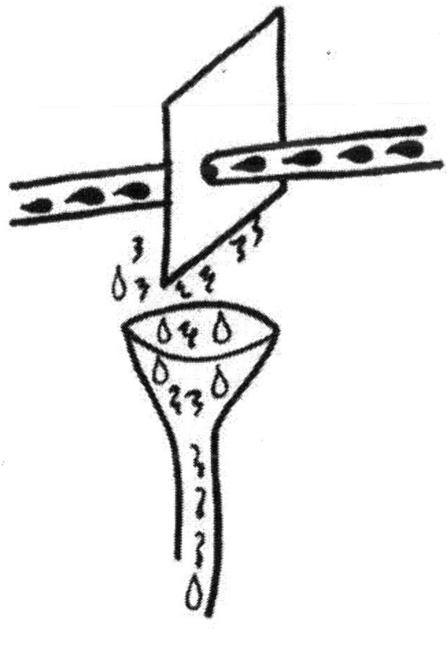

That is what our kidneys do. The entire blood circulation flows through the kidneys. Excess water is filtered out. That's why you pee right after you drink. Further, that's why the color of urine gets lighter if you drink more. Waste products like urea are filtered out. Any excess electrolytes and sugar are flushed out in that flow which we call urine.

Anatomy of the Genito-Urinary System
(continued)

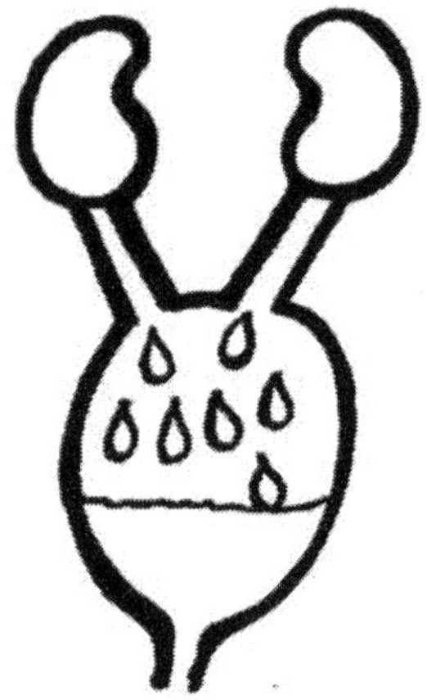

The two kidneys drain urine into the bladder through two tubes called ureters. The bladder holds urine until appropriate bathroom breaks.

The bladder is like a balloon. As it fills up it stretches. More stretch means more forceful ejection of the contents – just like a balloon.

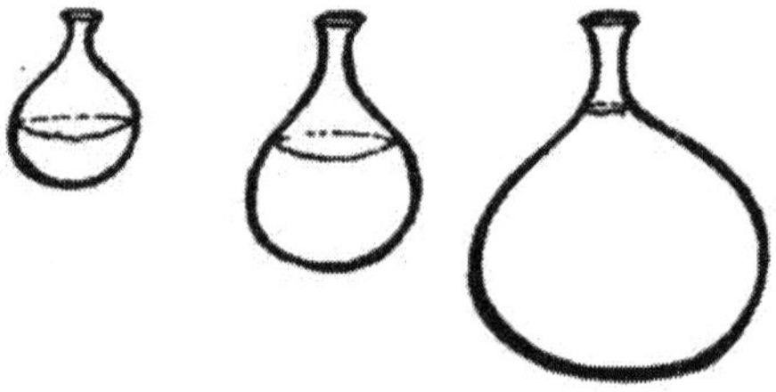

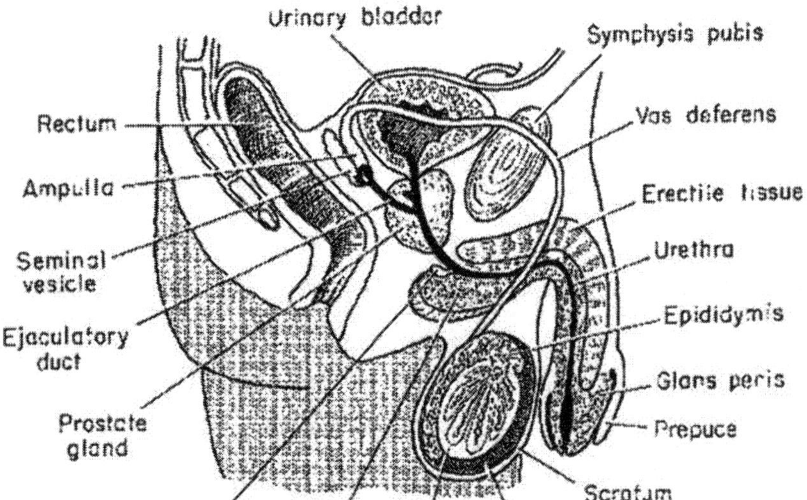

Urine leaves the bottom of the bladder through a tube called the urethra. Urine enters the urethra when the neck of the bladder relaxes. Emptying the bladder is under voluntary and involuntary control. If those terms are not familiar to you, just wait. They will be. Up to this point the male and female anatomy is the same.

In women the urethra is a short tube only about one inch from the bladder to its external orifice, the meatus. That is pronounced "mee-ah-tus", not "meat-us."

Anatomy of the Genito-Urinary System
(continued)

In males the reproductive organs connect to the urinary system here. Hence the name: *genito*-urinary system. In men the urethra leaves the bladder and extends to its orifice on the tip of the penis, the meatus.

Sperm is manufactured in the testes and stored in the epidydimi (plural of epidydimus). About 64 days elapse until the newly formed sperm matures. From the epidydimi the sperm continues to travel through the two tubes called the vas deferens.The two vas deferens connect to the urethra at the ejaculatory ducts. It is significant that following a vasectomy the two vas deferens are not clean of sperm for another 20-30 ejaculations.

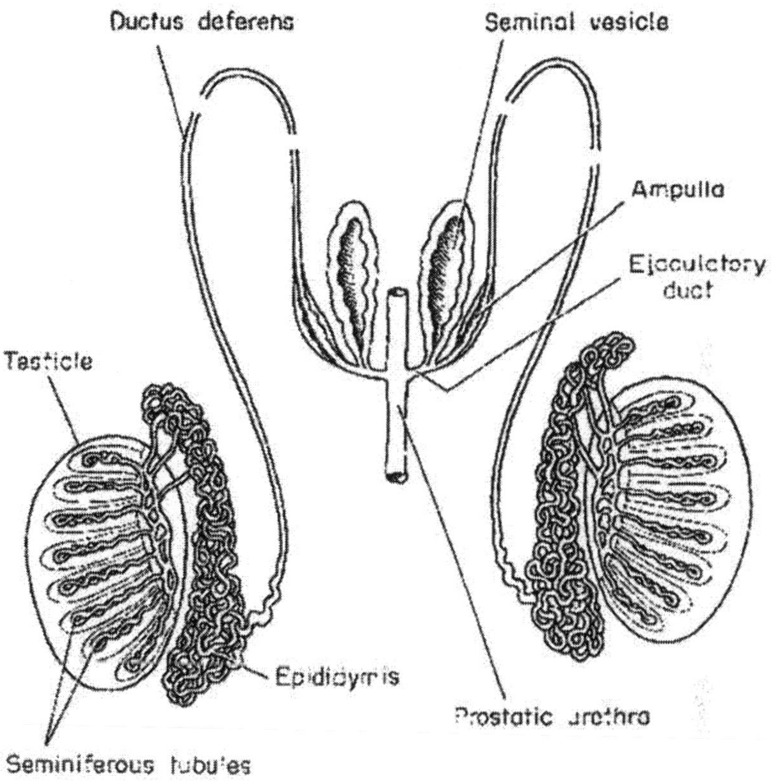

Also at this point another tube enters the urethra, the seminal vesicle. The volume of sperm is not enough to make the long journey from the penis through the vagina, cervix and uterus to the fallopian tube to meet the egg. Sperm is about 5% of the total ejaculate content. 95% of ejaculate is semen. Semen is produced in the seminal vesicles. It is a liquid largely composed of water, fructose and nutrients.

Below the neck of the bladder, surrounding the urethra is the walnut sized, prostate gland. Its purpose is to provide more seminal fluid.

Anatomy of the Genito-Urinary System

(continued)

To forcefully eject the semen and sperm mixture forward through the penis, the vas deferens contracts, the prostate gland closes around the urethra, and pelvic floor muscles contract rhythmically.

The closed prostrate gland does not allow the sperm and seminal fluid to flow backward toward the bladder. It also does not allow urine to flow during ejaculation.

That was an overview of the genito-urinary system. It did not cover the erection. The next few pages will explain how an erection happens.

An erection is when the penis is engorged with blood. The pudendal artery supplies blood to the penis. How the pudendal artery expands to supply more blood will be the subject of our next section.

Anatomy of the Penis and the Blood Flow for an Erection

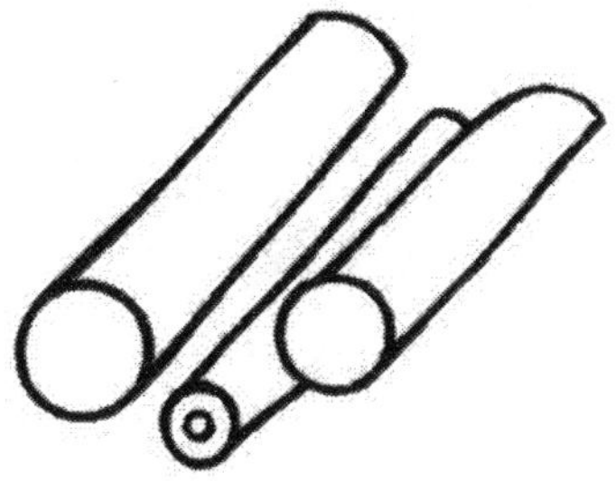

You probably already know that an erection is caused by blood filling the penis. So our explanation will go from there. The penis has three tubes two corpora cavernosa and one corpus spongeosum.

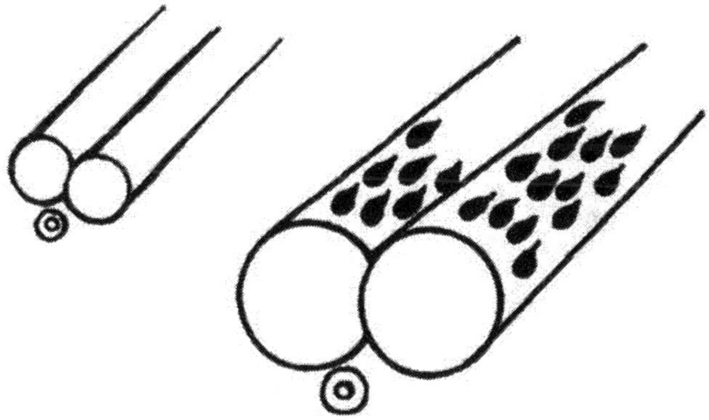

The corpora spongeosum houses the urethra. The urethra is the tube that connects to the bladder for purposes of urinating.

The two corpora cavernosa fill with blood to expand and lengthen to increase the size and stiffness of the penis.

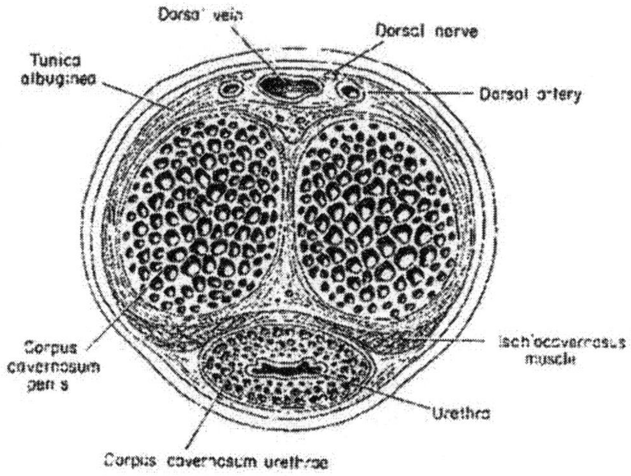

The blood flow to the penis is supplied by the pudendal artery. The pudendal artery provides blood for an erection. It supplies blood to the corpora cavernosa. The increased blood flow to the cavernosa is due to an increase of the pudendal artery's diameter. Most of this book will be about the physiology, pathophysiology and pharmacology of the pudendal artery.

Anatomy of the Penis and the Blood Flow for an Erection
(continued)

Just as the arteries provide oxygenated blood from the heart and lungs, veins return blood to the heart and lungs. Anyone who has ever had their blood drawn knows how easy it is to occlude venous blood flow. Just look at the bulging engorged veins after the phlebotomist tightens a tournaquette around your arm. The expanding corpora have a similar effect on the venous blood return from the penis.

The venous outflow is occluded by the expanding corpora which further increases the pressure. The pressure reaches about 100 mm Hg which raises the penis from the dependent position to the erect state. This is called the full erection phase

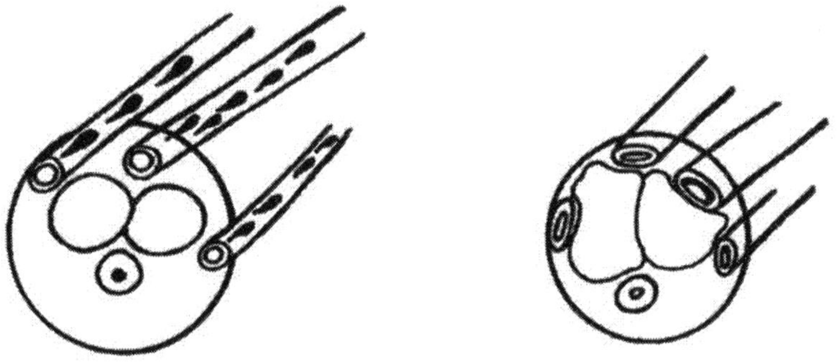

The ischio-cavernous and bulbo-cavernous muscles around the corpora cavernosa contract and further compress the penile veins to increase the pressure to several hundred mm Hg. Keep in mind the normal systolic blood pressure is only about 130 mm Hg.

The pressure in the glans (the extension of the corpora spongiosum to the tip of the penis) is about 1/3 the pressure in the corpora. This makes the tip of the penis softer which minimizes trauma to the female genitalia.

Physiology of Expanding Pudental Artery
(where the extra blood comes from)

On the last few pages we described the individual parts of a penis and how they enlarge and lengthen to bring about an erection. Now we will see how the artery expands in diameter to provide the extra blood to "pump up" the penis.

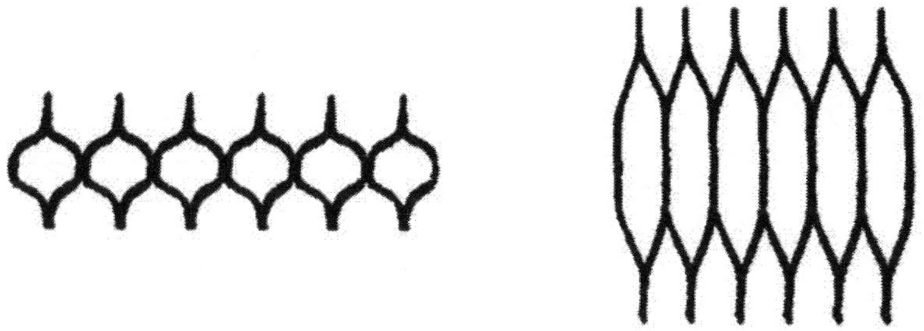

All arteries are surrounded by muscle cells. More specifically arteries are surrounded by smooth muscle. This gives any artery the ability to expand and deliver more blood as the body's needs change. Arteries increase in diameter by relaxation of the smooth muscle cells which surround them.

That is the most central fact of this book. All medications that pertain to erections depend on this fact: **Smooth muscle cells relax and the diameter of the artery increases, and blood flow increases.**

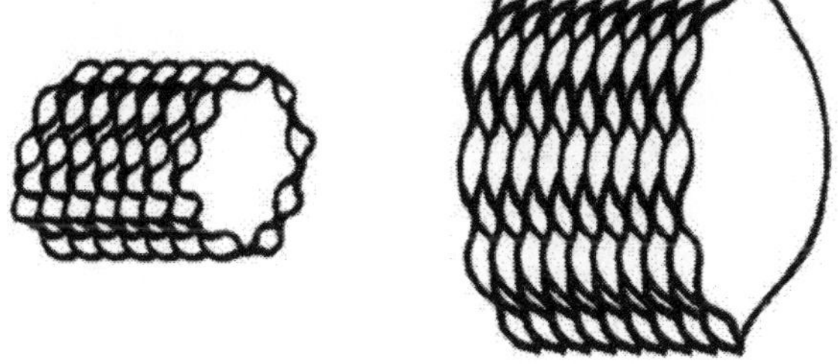

The diameter of the artery decreases when smooth muscle contracts. There are thousands of tiny muscles on every inch of artery.

Physiology of Expanding Pudental Artery
(continued)

Let's look at an individual smooth muscle cell.
Each muscle cell contracts when calcium enters the cell.

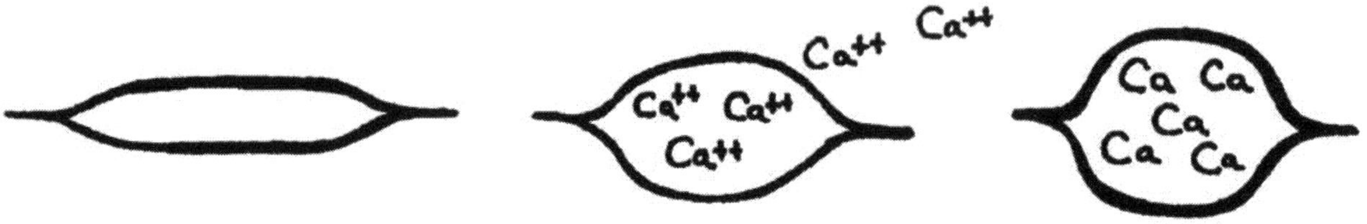

More calcium means more contraction.

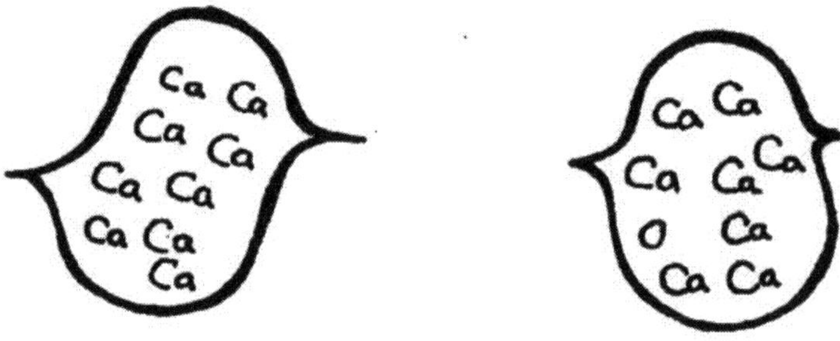

Calcium enters the cell through a calcium channel.

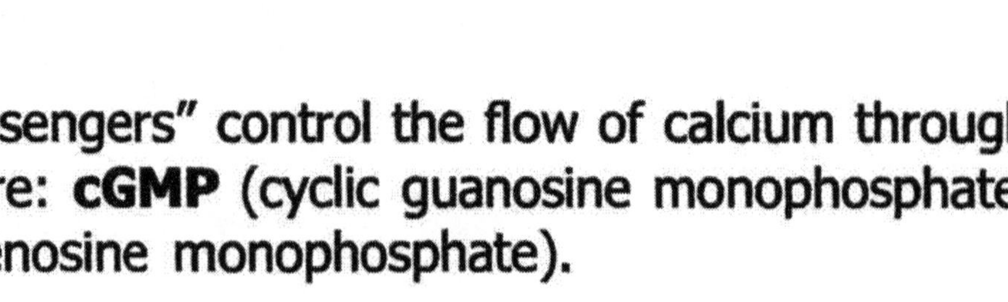

Two "second messengers" control the flow of calcium through the channel. They are: **cGMP** (cyclic guanosine monophosphate) and **cAMP** (cyclic adenosine monophosphate).

Physiology of Expanding Pudental Artery
(continued)

Each muscle cell has two types of nerves connected to it. One tells the cell to contract (which causes a flacid penis) and another tells the cell to relax (which causes an erect penis).

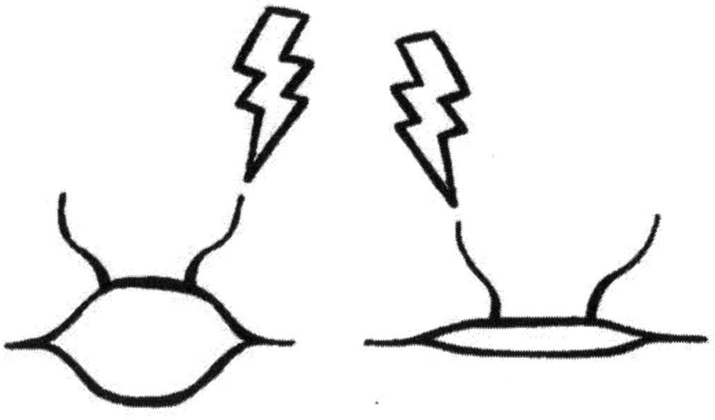

The nerve telling the cell to contract is called sympathetic and the nerve telling the cell to relax is called parasympathetic.

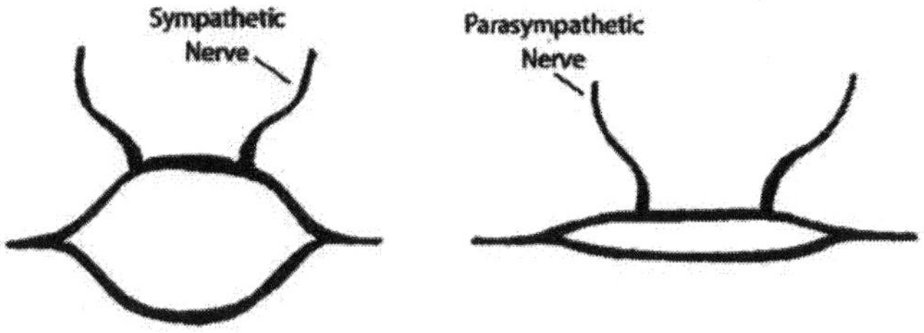

The parasympathetic (relax) nerve gets the muscle to relax by shooting a burst of nitric oxide to the cell.

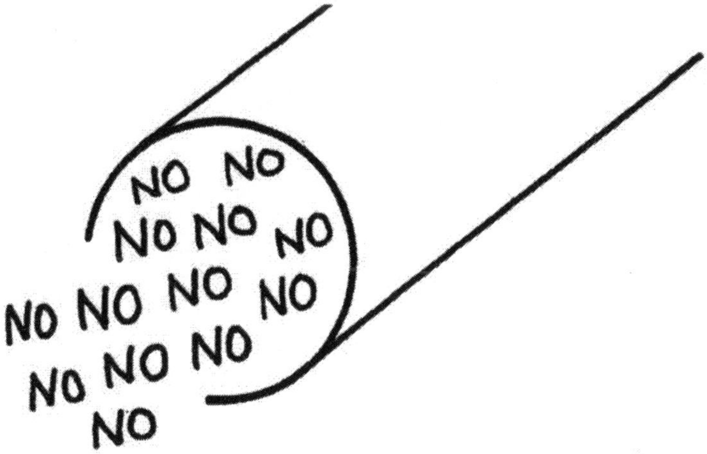

The sympathetic nerve gets the muscle to contract by shooting a burst of norepinepherine.

Physiology of Expanding Pudental Artery
(continued)

Nitric oxide is the "first messenger." Nitric oxide tells the "second messenger" cGmp to plug up the calcium channel. No calcium can enter the cells surrounding the pudendal artery and they can relax. The diameter increases. More blood flows into the penis and it becomes erect.

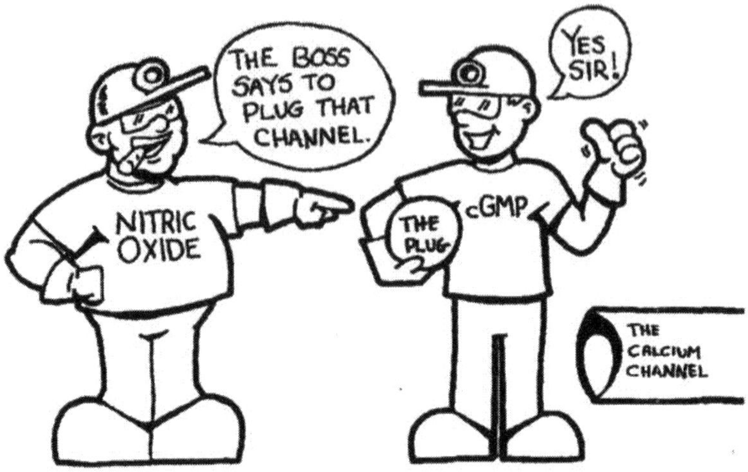

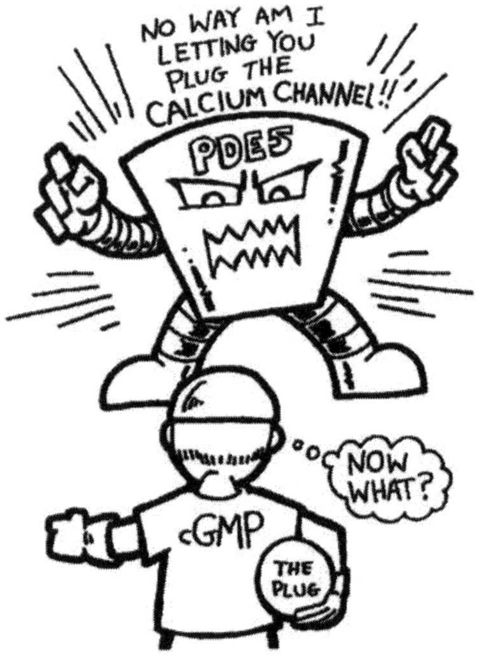

To moderate things, and keep men from walking around all day with an erection is phosphodiesterase (PDE). PDEs are found throughout the body. PDE_5 is found predominantly in the penis, which is what the oral PDE inhibitors block.

PDE_5 stops cGMP from plugging the calcium channel. More calcium enter the cell. All the muscle cells contract around the artery. The diameter of the artery decreases. Blood flow to the corpora slows. The penis becomes flaccid.

Physiology of Expanding Pudental Artery
(continued)

That is how phosphodiesterase limits erections. You may remember that Viagra®, Cialis®, and Levitra® are phosphodiesterase inhibitors. They **inhibit** phosphodiesterase, namely PDE_5. They help establish and maintain erections by "inhibiting" phosphodiesterase from stopping the second messenger as it tries to plug the calcium channel. I know that is confusing. Pictures show it better than words.

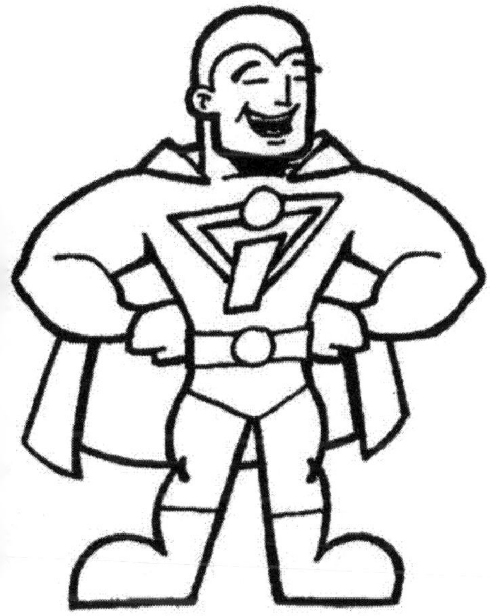

We have a new character, The Inhibitor.

The Inhibitor is flying through the blood stream and sees phosphdiesterase stopping cGMP plug the calcium channel.

He lands on the pudendal artery...

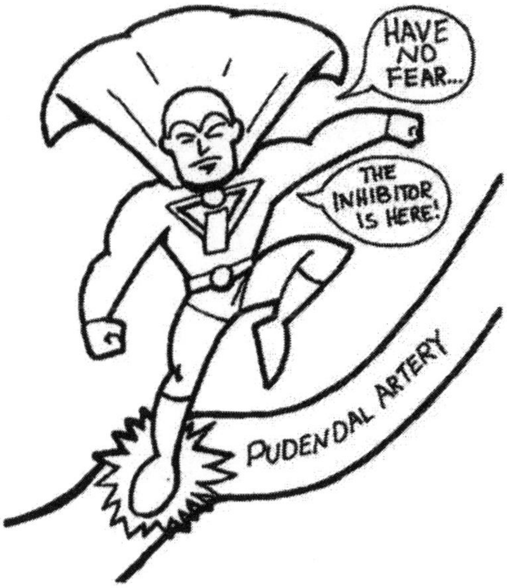

Physiology of Expanding Pudental Artery
(continued)

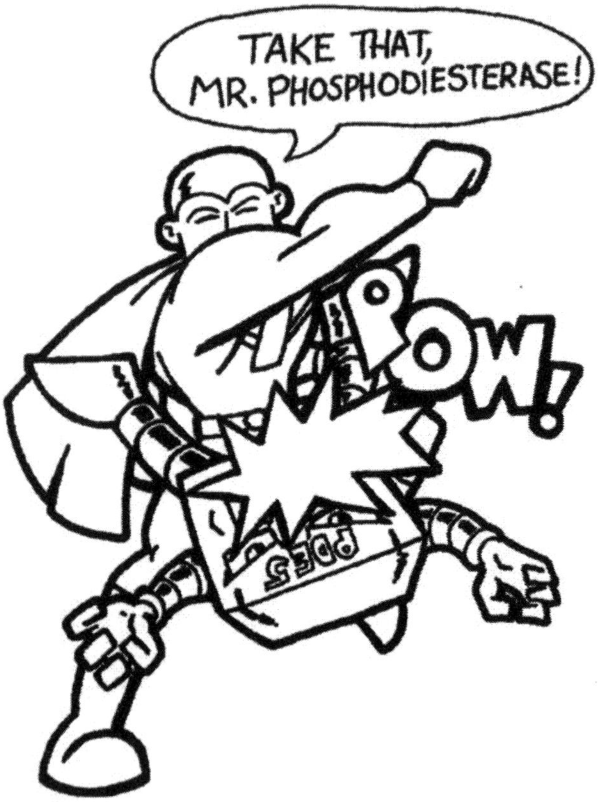

and he tells phosphodiesterase to get out of there

so cGmp can plug up the calcium channel. Now we have an erection.

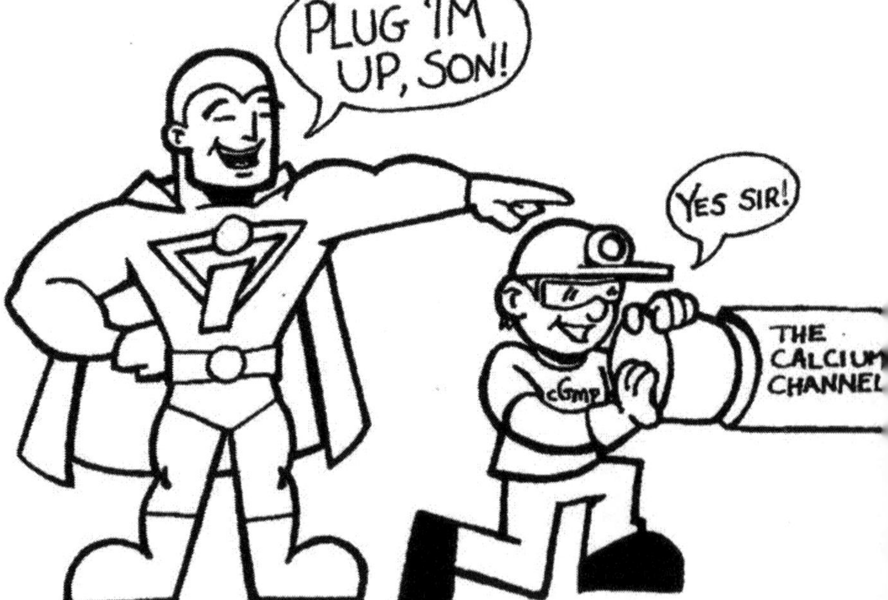

Flaccid Again

In our last exciting episode, the parasympathetic nerve was pouring nitric oxide into the the pudendal artery, cAMP was plugging the calcium channel, the smooth muscle cells were relaxing, blood flowed into the corpora, in other words, an erection. That's where we left off.

Then the sympathetic nervous system takes over. All the muscles surrounding the vas deferens and the seminal fluid ducts and the prostrate gland forcefully contract to ejaculate sperm. Norepinepherine (you'll learn about this on the next page) initiates sympathetic contraction of smooth muscles. The muscle cells surrounding the pudendal artery also contract which reduces the blood blow to the corpora and ends the erection.

That was a quick look at one type of medication which promote erections. We explained phosphodiesterase inhibitors, Viagra®, Cialis® and Levitra®. There are other medications to promote erections. Since you are familiar with the cartoon characters we will continue the explanation with the same characters.

Three More Medications

The next three medications we will look at are phentolamine, alprostadil and papaverine. If Viagra®, Cialis® or Levitra® do not work any of these or all of them combined would likely be the next step.

The next medication we will look at is Phentolamine. Phentolamine is an alpha one blocker.

You may remember there are two nerves attached to each muscle cell. We talked about the parasympathetic nerve which stimulates erections. There is also the sympathetic nerve which stops an erection. To stop an erection, sympathetic nerve emits its own "first messenger", norepinepherine.

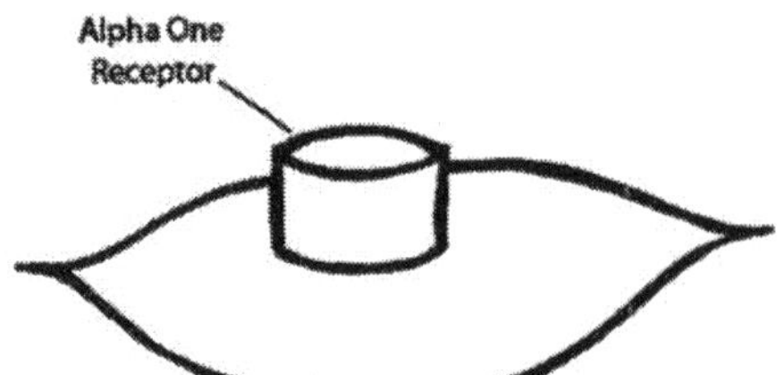

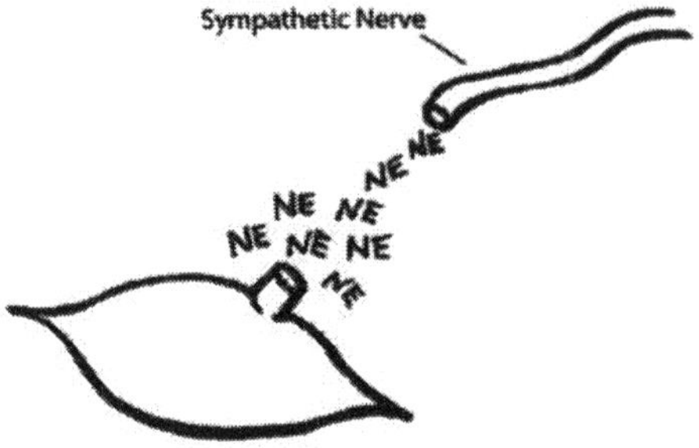

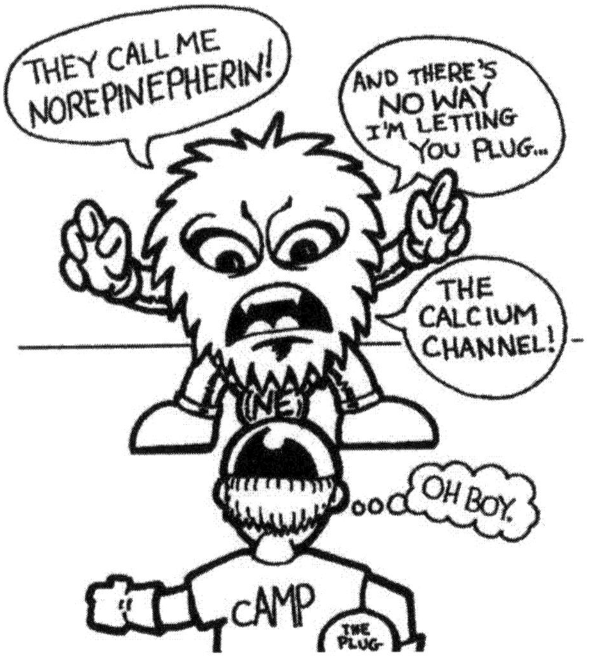

Norepinepherine enters the muscle cell through a door called an alpha one receptor.

Three More Medications
(continued)

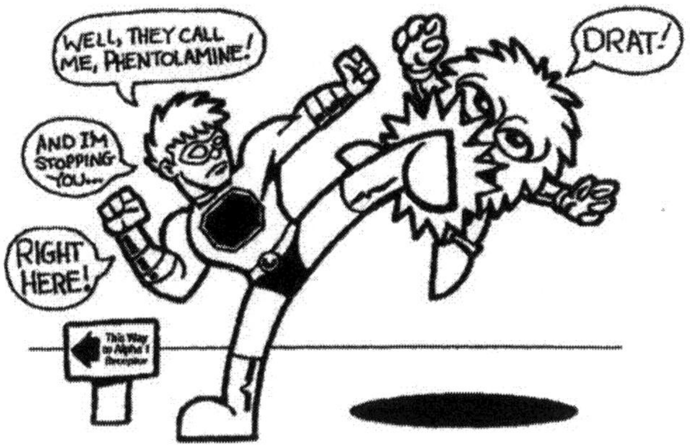

Norepinepherine can be stopped right where it enters the muscle cell, at the alpha one receptor. Phentolamine stops the norepinepherine from reaching the muscle cell. Now the parasympathetic surge is stronger which promotes an erection.

The next medication is alprostadil. The generic name is prostaglandin E_1. You can see the word "prostate" in the name.

In the 1930's these messengers were first isolated from prostrate gland tissue. It is abbreviated PGE_1. PGE_1 tells cAMP to plug the calcium channel thereby stimulating an erection. PGE_1 has been synthesized into a medication called aprostadil. It can be injected by a very small diabetic needle or inserted into the urethra.

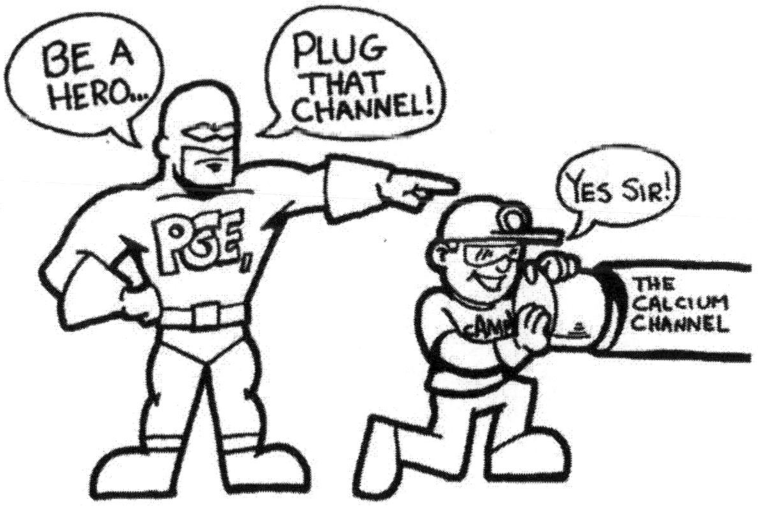

Three More Medications
(continued)

The third medication is papaverine. Papaverine is a nonspecific phosphdiesterase inhibitor. You remember that Viagra® is phosphodiesterase-5 inhibitor. Papaverine inhibits more kinds of phosphodiesterase. It inhibits phosphodiesterase-2, 3 and 4 (PDE_2, PDE_3, PDE_4). Papaverine enhances the action of both cGMP and cAMP by blocking those three types of phosphodiesterase.

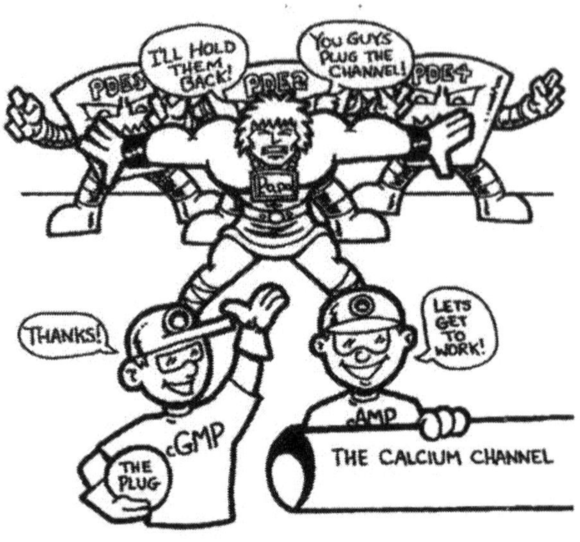

These medications are given by injection, self injection into the corpus cavernosa. The needle is very small, an insulin or tuberculin needle. That size needle causes no pain. Ask any insulin dependent diabetic. The two copora cavernosas are located at 3 o'clock and 9 o'clock on the penile shaft. The injections should alternate from side to side. (The 12 o'clock position must be avoided because of the arteries and nerves as well as the 6 o'clock position due to the urethra. Men on blood thinners should use caution as this may cause a hematoma or bruise.) Aprostadil also comes in the form of an intraurethral pellet wih an applicator.

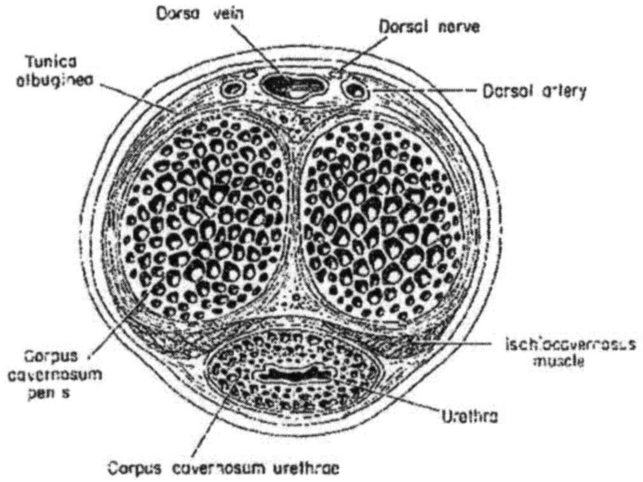

These injectable medications tend to produce a firmer erection than the oral medications. However, due to the invasive nature of delivery, They are usually offered if the oral medications have failed.

Most frequent causes for erectile dysfunction

Loss of the ability to achieve an erection may be due to any of the following reasons:

- **Vascular damage to the pudendal artery.** This is usually caused by high blood pressure, high cholesterol, smoking and aging.

- **Medications**, particularly high blood pressure medications

- **Psychological issues** are another cause. This book cannot begin to cover the brain-penis connection. On this book's level of explanation, I can't say it better than the following joke, which is serious:
  The most important sex organ in humans is between the ears.

- The third reason is **prostate surgery**. Nerves, which control smooth muscle, can be damaged.

- A fourth reason is **low Testosterone levels.**

Any combination of these would cause loss of the ability to achieve an erection.

Costs

The three oral medications typically cost between 10 and 20 dollars a tablet. Insurance coverage is minimal. To save money, it may be possible to achieve the desired effect with 1/2 tablet. The lowest effective does should be used to minimize side effects and undesired prolonged erection (priapism).

Other Options

The next two options may be used with oral medications or separately.

Elastic Ring

The elastic ring may be used to augment medication or may be used seperately. Once an erection has been attained the the ring maintains it by occluding venous blood return from the corpora.

Vacuum Device

The vacuum device is a cylinder is a cylinder slightly bigger than the penis. An attached pump creates a vacuum around the penis. Into this low pressure space blood fills the penis, in paticular the corpora. That is of course an erection. To augment this, a elastic ring may be put in place beforehand. There are many hand operated and batter operated systems.

The cost is between $30 and $500. They may be purchased from medical suppliers with a prescription or for adult video and sex supply stores or the internet without a prescription.

The last option is **surgery**.

Nitrates

If you have seen the Viagra® advertisements they say not to take Viagra if you are taking nitroglycerine for chest pain. Let me say that in other words:

Viagra®, Cialis® & Levitra® are absolutely contra-indicated for men taking nitrates (oral, sublingual or topical). Do not take Viagra®, Cialis® or Levitra® if you are taking any nitrates.

The reason is that nitroglycerine turns into nitric oxide. You may remember that nitric oxide leads to dilating the vasculature. Combined, the two medications could cause a loss of blood pressure that could be fatal.

....on the subject of warnings in bold letters:

MEN WITH ERECTILE DYSFUNCTION ARE AT HIGHER RISK FOR HEART ATTACKS

Whether or not you chose to pursue medication to treat erectile dysfunction, tell your doctor about the condition. If your doctor has any questions about why you are bringing up this subject, tear this page out and bring it with you.

Herbal Male Enhancement

There are many, many over-the-counter medications which are not approved by the Food and Drug Administration. That is to say, there have not been any controlled studies to show any benefit from any of the ingredients.

You will also see many newspaper articles about PDE inhibitors illegally added to those herbal medications.

Our recommendation is to use only FDA approved medications under the direction of a physician.

Seeing a Urologist

Usually the first visit would be to discuss the diagnosis and treatment, draw blood and get a prescription.

Blood test would include:
- HbA_{1c}
- Cholesterol
- Testosterone
- PSA

These are checked as abnormalities may be a contributing cause to the erectile dysfunction.

Prostrate Specific Antigen (PSA) would be tested if you are over 50 years old, have a history of prostrate problems, or are African-American and over 40 years old. Elevated cholesterol levels can suggest arterial damage. An elevated HbA1c can indicate diabetes even if the blood sugar is normal. Testosterone affects libido and low levels can cause erectile dysfunction.

A follow up appointment would be in order for a change of medications if the first prescription doesn't work. We have discussed the second round of medications is the oral phosphodiesterases don't work. That said, there are minor differences between Viagra®, Cialis® and Levitra®. It is possible that one of them may work where another failed. More tests may be recommended.

Claims by Medical Doctors with Large Newspaper Ads

You will see in newspapers large advertisements by medical doctors which claim sexual fulfillment. They usually show an attractive couple in some level of physical intimacy. The subtle or not so subtle suggestion is that you can achieve that by purchasing their services.

Be wary of such claims.

There is no FDA approved medication, treatment or test available to them which can not be obtained from any urologist in any office big or small, pretentious or plain. The training and accreditation of any board certified urologist in this country is identical.

Alcohol & Relaxation

You may remember the word parasympathetic nervous system on Page 14. An erection is one of many forms of the parasympathetic nervous system in action. A state of relaxation would facilitate all of the parasympathetic actions.

Anything in the direction of relaxation would favor an erection.

Small amounts of alcohol which induce relaxation stimulate an erection. Small amounts of alcohol are vasodilatory. We know about dilating the pudendal artery.

Large amounts of alcohol suppress the central nervous system which in-turn suppresses erections.

Long term alcohol consumption also damages liver function which decreases testosterone production.

Cigarettes

Cigarette smoking causes vascular damage. You already know cigarette smoking is a major risk factor for heart attacks. Cigarettes have the same effect on the coronary arteries as they do on the pudendal artery: the smooth lining of the blood vessels is damaged.

Other vascular risk factors that can damage the pudental artery include hypertension, high cholesterol, and diabetes. It is worth noting that a man with erectile dysfunction had double the likelihood of a heart attack.

Negative Side Effects

The most common side effect of phosphodiesterase inhibitors is headache. Others include back pain, vision and hearing changes.

Priapism

The advertisements for Viagra®, Levitra® and Cialis® talk about a painful erection lasting more than four hours. That is called priapism. They rarely occur. Should it happen call your doctor or go to the emergency room. The most frequent cure for priapism is an injection of a sympathetic stimulant to override the parasympathetic action (but you already knew that!).

About the authors

Malcolm Rosenberg, RN began his career as a nurse and nurse educator after receiving his Associates Degree from Broward Community College in 1989. Since he wanted his students to understand the content without being overly concerned with note taking, he put together handouts for the students of exactly what was on the overhead projector. Those packages then became these books.

Ralph Zagha attended Foster City Elementary school where he showed promise in coloring and baseball. Because his last name started with a "Z" he was always seated in the last row. Being out of range of his teacher's watchful eye gave him the opportunity to shoot spitballs. He also attended the University of California San Diego with a major in chemistry/ biochemistry, Tufts University School of Medicine followed by a Urology residency at Harvard & Tufts teaching hospitals, Massachussets General Hospital, Lahey Clinic and Boston Childrens Hospital.

Dr. Zagha has lived up to early expectations: he continues to excel at coloring and baseball. Since his name still begins with a "Z" he continues to get seated in the last row of American Medical Association Conventions where he continues to shoot spitballs. He is happily married to Stacy and the father of a wonderful young son, Mark.

and the illustrator

Christopher Saghy is a graphic designer by day, dad by night and an artist every moment in between. A cartoonist at heart, Chris has never lost his love of drawing funny pictures, even when he is in full fantasy art mode. He believes art, as well as life in general should be fun and injects almost all his work with his slightly off-kilter humor.

Chris lives in Frizzellburg, Maryland with his wife Kathy, daughter Shannon, son Michael and a very large cat named Figasaurus. His fantasy and comic art can be viewed on the web by googling Christopher Saghy.

For Students...For L.P.N.s...For R.N.s...

VIAGRA SIMPLIFIED
UNDERSTANDING THE ERECTION

by MALCOLM ROSENBERG, R.N.

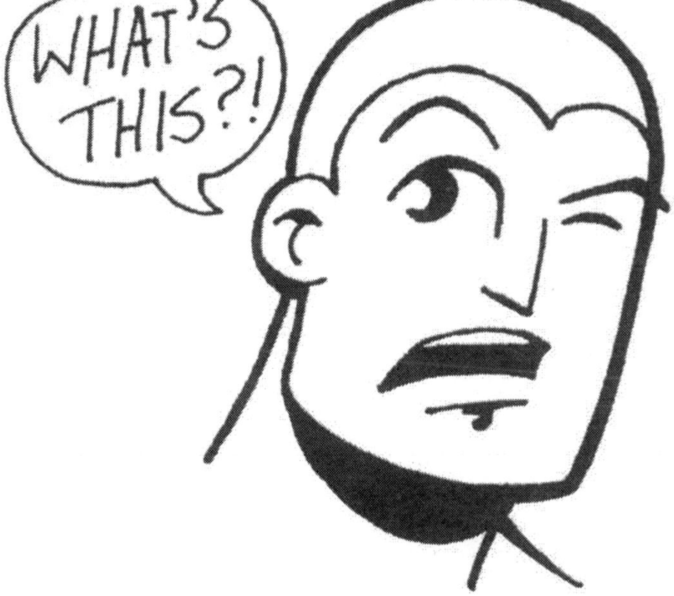

- *HOW AN ERECTION WORKS*
- *WHY PROBLEMS OCCUR*
- *HOW MEDICATION & TREATMENT CAN HELP*

MORE GREAT BOOKS!

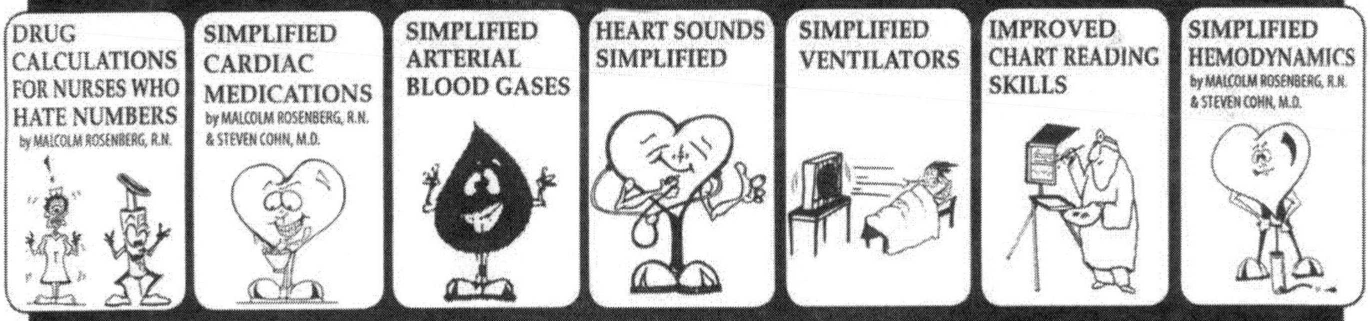

To get more information and order online: **www.simplifiednursing.com**
or send a check or money order made out to:
Malcolm Rosenberg • P.O. Box 770793 • Coral Springs, FL 33077 • (954) 753-5915

NAME________________________ E-MAIL________________

ADDRESS____

CITY____________________ STATE________ ZIP________________

- Simplified Viagra .... $??? ☐
- Drug Calculations For Nurses Who Hate Numbers .... $18.95 ☐
- Simplified Cardiac Medications .... $18.95 ☐
- Simplified Arterial Blood Gases .... $18.95 ☐
- Hemodynamics .... $11.95 ☐
- Simplified Ventilators .... $7.95 ☐
- Heart Sounds Simplified .... $7.95 ☐
- Simplified Blood Clotting .... $6.95 ☐
- Improved Chart Reading Skills .... $3.95 ☐

Best Value
Get All 9 Books for $??.00

TOTAL ENCLOSED $ __________

For more infomation write or call:

MALCOLM ROSENBERG
P.O. BOX 770793
CORAL SPRINGS, FL 33077
(954) 753-5915

and PLEASE VISIT OUR WEBSITE AT:
www.simplifiednursing.com

Viagra Simplified and Other ED Medications: Understanding The Erection ©2007 Retail: $7.95

ISBN 0-9725483-7-8
9780972548373
0 700814 498061
7 00814 49806 1

Made in the USA
Monee, IL
05 November 2026

68020859R00020